# The Silver Water Coincidences

Will a unique form of nanosilver ever be an
approved treatment for cancer, TB, HIV and
several less serious conditions?

Dan McAneny

*For Harry Watson,*
*who wanted to save as many lives as he could…*
*and where he couldn't, reduce pain and suffering*

# The Silver Water
# Coincidences

# Table of Contents

# From the Author to the Reader

This is an updated version of the original book published in 2014. As of this writing, it is 2019. Harry passed earlier this year at age 96, and although he never made any claims for nanosilver, he told me a week before he died that he personally felt he had added 12 years to his life by using it plus baking soda and sometimes drinking a special water. That's just his belief, of course, and no one associated with Precious Waters™ makes any claims about Harry or anyone else mentioned in this book.

Rod Stroope, who contributed so much to the original version, is no longer associated with Precious Waters Inc. After Harry's passing, his wife Donna happily transferred the distribution rights and the right to use the name Precious Waters™ to Susan Marie and Mark Szehner. Donna has known Susan Marie ever since her husband used the "silver water" as described in the second chapter ("Vietnam Vet Cheats Death from Bacterial Lung Infection.")

Like Harry did after his first cancer was beaten back at age 85, Susan's husband stopped taking the nanosilver. When other cancers later occurred, he decided not to take any treatment, and died in a matter of months. That did not lessen Susan's enthusiasm for Precious Waters™

nanosilver, and she was eager to carry on Harry's legacy. She and Mark formed Trinity Silver Solutions, which is now the distributor for Precious Waters™ products. They operate the website, which is where people can order if they like at <u>PreciousWatersInc.com</u>. Susan also encourages people to call her or Mark just as they called Harry. The number is 530-739-8600, and it is printed on the label.

The product is also available in gel form, and Susan suggested including in this introduction that if the gel stops spraying, it is usually possible to remove the top, pour a bit of liquid nanosilver into the bottle, shake it a bit, and it will extend the time the gel sprays easily.

The original introduction from 2014 is included after this one. There are two important points made there that should be expanded and reinforced at this time. First, some people concluded that, despite the repeated statement that no claims are made, there is an implied promise that Precious Waters™ nanosilver will help cure a variety of illnesses. **No one should ever purchase it thinking it will help cure any condition. It is sold only as a dietary supplement, nothing else. There are no implied promises about anything!**

The placebo effect is firmly established in medical literature. It could well be that people taking nanosilver also develop a strong belief that their condition, whatever it is, will be healed. It is entirely possible that their beliefs alone were the major factor in their recovery. Also, in many cases, people were also taking chemotherapy or a prescription drug that was the cause for their recovery,

b

and it is quite possible that nanosilver had no effects whatsoever. Further, just because one person with a particular condition experiences recovery for whatever reason, that does not mean another person with the same condition will experience any positive results.

The second point refers to the question posed on the cover, as to whether a unique form of nanosilver will ever be an approved treatment for cancer and other serious illnesses. **At this point the answer apparently is a firm NO!**

At the time the original version of this book was published, there was hope on Harry's part that doctors might want to conduct some trials that would show it could be effective in these cases. Experience over the past four years indicates that doctors generally do not want their patients taking nanosilver while they are being treated with chemotherapy, prescription drugs or any other treatment they might be administering. That applies not only to major illnesses, but minor ones as well.

All of the stories in the original version, Chapters 1 through 12, are told as they were four years ago, with an occasional update. Some stories that were included in my blog between 2014 and 2017 are added in two additional chapters. After 2017 the focus of my writing changed to other subjects, and I stopped keeping track of stories.

The former chapters 13, 14 and 15 are now chapters 15, 16 and 17. The new Chapter 16, which gives label information, has been updated to show the name and address for Trinity Silver Solutions. The new Chapter 13 includes some 2014 stories from my blog that were not included in the original version and others from 2015 to 2017 after the book was published. The new Chapter 14 includes a few stories from Harry's family about their experiences with the liquid and gel. They are included in keeping with Susan's emphasis on people taking it when they are experiencing less serious conditions which are common. Like Harry did, she points out that no claims are made for treating them or any more serious condition.

One final point made in the earlier version: I have no financial interest in Trinity Silver Solutions LLC or Precious Waters Inc., and make no money when people buy the product. My sole purpose in writing this book was to help Harry and Donna—and now Susan and Mark—to spread the word about these coincidences

**Original Introduction**

"Silver water" is what many people call Precious Waters™ brand nanosilver. As explained in this book, it is a unique, highly engineered form of nanosilver. Studies conducted in 2006 by scientists at Pennsylvania State University and Arizona State University documented the fact that Precious Waters™ nanosilver poses no harm when consumed.

Separate lab tests in 2007 conducted by others showed its effectiveness against HIV and Avian Influenza, and the fact that when it was combined with 19 different antibiotics, it improved their effectiveness. They also noted the safe use of silver as an orally consumed preventive agent, demonstrated and supported by reports from the EPA and the US Department of Health and

d

Human Services, where in a 76-week long study, dogs that inhaled silver showed activity in the lung in one hour, with 90% of the silver carried to the liver by the blood within six hours.

People frequently refer to this product as simply "Precious Waters," and to keep this book easy to read and consistent, I will use the term "Precious Waters™" to refer to the nanosilver in liquid form. When referring to the Topical Spray Gel, it will be noted as such.

The FDA allows Precious Waters™ to be sold only as a dietary supplement, when it was "grandfathered" in with health products such as vitamins and minerals for oral consumption as a dietary supplement. That means, while it has been rigorously tested in the lab for efficacy and safety, and while it conforms to DSHEA requirements under FDA guidelines, no claims can be made about its effectiveness in fighting any disease.

Harry Watson, the founder of Precious Waters, Inc., never makes any claims beyond those on the company's website at www.preciouswatersinc.com. As for me, my goal is simply to spread the word about this wonderful product because of its potential to help so many people. I make no money when people buy Precious Waters™ and have no financial interest in Harry's company.

While no claims can be made for the effectiveness of Precious Waters™ in the U.S., all of us do need to pay attention to the evidence that our physical senses provide. When Harry hears of wonderful things happening to people who take Precious Waters™, it is only natural to wonder whether it might be capable of fighting any number of diseases.

**Right now there is no proof that it is capable of fighting even one disease, nor are there any U.S. based clinical trials indicating that it is.** Perhaps in the future such trials will be conducted and claims can be made. But that is unlikely, because clinical trials in the United States take vast amounts of time and money, requiring the resources of a large corporation.

In the meantime, what are we to conclude when people take Precious Waters™ and, at the same time, experience dramatic improvement or full recovery from diseases ranging from cancer, TB and HIV, to lung disease, endometriosis, herpes simplex, and a number of less serious common illnesses? **Certainly not that it is a cure or that it treats any of these diseases in any way.** FDA regulations forbid a claim like that. As of now, in the United States, no one can indicate that there is any cause/effect relationship between the taking of Precious Waters™ and the improved physical conditions people report.

But here is what we can do. We can keep track of story after story where good things happen to people taking it. We can observe a *correlation* between taking this unique form of nanosilver and people's physical improvements, even if we cannot claim *causation*. When dozens of such stories pile up, we can observe an impressive number of coincidences in which many people get better at the same time they happen to be taking Precious Waters™, sometimes with baking soda and sometimes not, sometimes in combination with antibiotics

f

and sometimes not. There are a few anecdotes where people do not tell their doctors they are taking it. That should not be interpreted as recommending that anyone hold back information from treating physicians.

All I ask is that you read the stories and note the coincidences. If you have a condition that can be successfully treated with conventional drugs and/or surgery, it's probably wise to get those treatments as I did when I had cancer five different times, with excellent success each time. On the other hand, if doctors have told you or someone you know that there is nothing more that can be done, or that they don't know the cause of your illness and aren't able to cure it, then perhaps you might start looking into a variety of alternatives.

In my case, even though the chemo, radiation and surgery worked well, I also drank Essiac tea, ate a lot of broccoli, and got treated with Chinese acupuncture and herbs. Did any of them help? I don't know. I figured it wouldn't hurt to use them and I had nothing to lose. Likewise, Precious Waters™ nanosilver has been taken by hundreds of people with no ill effects to my knowledge, so I figured I had nothing to lose by taking it as a preventive, in the hope that it might help prevent future infections from viruses, bacteria or fungi.

Harry's main goal in making Precious Waters™ available to the public is to help people recover the way he did after taking it, but neither he nor his company will ever claim that this unique form of nanosilver treated or cured anything, in his case or in any of the "coincidences" reported in this book. For people with less serious

g

conditions, he suggests it will assist their immune system to help avoid opportunistic viruses and bacteria that frequently cause minor illnesses.

It should be noted that, besides Harry, the other person who has contributed substantially to making this nanosilver dietary supplement available and affordable is Rod Stroope, who has served for some time as CEO of Precious Waters, Inc., and who shares Harry's passion for helping as many people as possible, not just with major diseases, but with many common ailments as well.

One last note: silver has been known for centuries to fight infections, **including many that do not involve serious diseases. In fact, many of the coincidences noted in this book involve common conditions.** All of the stories in this book relate to people taking Precious Waters™ in liquid form internally, or the topical spray gel externally. Reported here are observations, interviews and research I've done related to Precious Waters™. I can offer no information or knowledge about other forms of nanosilver.

# Chapter 1:  The Story of Harry Watson

In 1999 Harry Watson learned he had prostate cancer. It was successfully treated by conventional means. Eight years later, he learned that the cancer had migrated to his abdomen. It was a very aggressive form of cancer—pseudomyxoma peritonei—associated with the production of mucous-like fluid. Doctors did what they could, but gave him only months to live.

With just one month to live according to their timetable, Harry started taking nanosilver, along with baking soda, and recovered quickly. When friends asked him to get some for them, he gave away his last bottle. When he started researching nanosilver on the internet for others who asked, he found it was very expensive from available sources. One family even paid $8000 for a bottle. Finally he located a manufacturer who could produce a unique form of nanosilver using proprietary processes resulting in a very high quality nanosilver, and later he identified a second such manufacturer. Harry is a global distributor, selling high quality nanosilver at an affordable price so most people can easily afford it.

Being an exceptionally energetic and robust individual, Harry assumed he was totally free of cancer and stopped taking the nanosilver. After all, he had been a

World War II fighter pilot, a captain on 747's and DC 10's for 32 years with Continental Airlines, and a youth league football coach from a tiny town in Texas who took his undersized team to California to win a championship. A doctor visiting from India warned him not to stop taking the nanosilver, but Harry was preoccupied with business matters, so he stopped taking it.

Harry's cancer came back with a vengeance a couple of years later, and when the doctors opened him up they drained him, sewed him back up, and declared he was not going to make it. One doctor who liked him came by to pay his respects, saying, "I'm sorry, but this is the last time I'll see you, Harry."

Harry's wife Donna tried to tell the head oncologist about nanosilver and "the power of prayer," but the doctor would have none of it. He quickly brushed her comments aside with, "I'm the expert here. Listen to me." He gave Harry a short time to live. Harry once again researched his cancer on the internet and found that the only conventional treatments suggested were still very harsh, with little chance of success.

Very sick at this point, with terrible pain, coughing, and tightening of the abdominal muscles, Harry started taking Precious Waters™ again, one ounce three times a day with a teaspoon of baking soda. Amazingly, on the morning of the fourth day, he woke with no pain. In a few weeks he felt totally better and got back to work full-time! Harry is now 92, and as energetic as ever. He still takes a small amount of nanosilver daily.

Precious Waters™ is essentially nano-sized particles

2

of pure silver in purified water that have undergone processing at the manufacturer. They have a uniquely high surface area to mass ratio and a specific positive electrical charge. Unlike traditional colloidal silver, it is not in ionic form before consumption, and does not stay in the system or lead to argyria, a discoloration of the skin. If you were to pour some into a shot glass, for instance, it would look just like water, and would taste that way when you drank it. You would not see the particles, since they are so tiny they are not visible to the naked eye. That's why people commonly call it "silver water."

The particles are evenly distributed throughout the purified water solution at a concentration of 10 parts per million. The silver particles are highly bio-available, meaning they disassociate from the water quickly, and they are bio-active, meaning they pass across the cell membrane readily to fully neutralize the pathogen.

Through contacts in Africa, Harry has made Precious Waters™ available in Kenya. Harry and I recently spoke with Joseph Muriethi, who has been involved in two clinical trials conducted there in 2011 and 2012. Mr. Muriethi holds a degree in Nursing from the highly regarded National University in San Diego CA. He administers treatments directly to patients in these trials, and confirmed that several doctors were involved in each of the trials, which were carefully controlled and monitored.

The first was conducted on 45 patients with HIV, cancer, diabetes, hypertension, malaria and other diseases.

The rate of improvement or cure was 83%. The second trial, conducted by doctors who used Precious Waters™ along with three drugs, was 50% funded by the Kenyan government. It included 100 patients with HIV, cancer, diabetes, hypertension, fibroids and dermatological conditions. The rate of improvement or cure was 94%.

The results were so remarkable that the government initially indicated it might fund part of a larger trial involving 5000 patients, but there has been a change in government, and potential funding is still being considered.

There are no anecdotes about Precious Waters™ being taken by people in the U.S, who had either diabetes or hypertension (high blood pressure), so Harry and I questioned Mr. Muriethi about participants in the Kenya trials who had those conditions. He stated that all the people with hypertension improved, and seven of them no longer needed to take blood pressure medication. There were between 15 and 20 patients in these trials with diabetes. They improved to varying degrees. Some who had taken medication as often as 3 times a day, he said, were able to reduce that to once a week or even less, as needed.

## Chapter 2: Vietnam Vet Cheats Death from Bacterial Lung Infection

This is the story of Bill, a Vietnam vet in his sixties, living in the Fullerton CA area. Bill's wife Susan rushed Bill to the hospital in September of 2013, with pain in his groin. He was diagnosed with a bladder infection and sent home. Bill was put on Levofloxacin, a strong antibiotic, for two weeks. He remained ill through October, and could barely walk by the end of the month. He went to work, but could only lie on a couch after work, lacking the energy to do anything else.

In early November, he passed out in a bathroom and hit his head on the floor. On November 11, his primary care doctor insisted he get a chest X-ray on the way home. The X-ray showed that his lungs were black and that he most likely had TB. He was instructed to go to the hospital immediately. The technicians would not let Susan and Bill leave without masks, as Bill was considered contagious.

Bill spent five days in the hospital. He was diagnosed with the rare Bullae Lung Disease. His pulmonary doctor said he had seen only eight cases of Bullae Lung Disease in 39 years of practice. The disease causes large bubbles (Bullae is French for bubble) to form in the lungs, making it difficult to expel air completely.

To complicate matters even more, one large bubble (the size of a man's clenched fist) and several smaller ones were filled with pus. The doctors wanted to perform a biopsy to determine the bacterial source but were concerned that the pus infection might spill out and migrate to other parts of Bill's body. By the end of day one, the only solution on the table was to remove his infected left lung.

It should be noted that Bill was exposed to Agent Orange in Vietnam as the pilot of a Medevac rescue helicopter, and ran a woodworking business in San Diego County for 15 years where he was exposed to fumes from stains and varnishes, and to a lot of wood dust. He also worked in an industry for a number of years that generated paper dust. In addition, the air where Bill lived was of poor quality, with particle smog blowing back and forth overhead. There were several possible contributors to the source of his lung disease.

Bill soon became the talk of the hospital. Several doctors were amazed that anyone could have such an advanced infection and life-threatening lung disease … *and not know he even had it until the day he walked in the door.* As you might expect, there were many visitors to his room, all curious to see this phenomenon.

On the second day, the hospital's top surgeon, an Iraq vet, minced no words with Bill. After assuring him that he was the best surgeon for this type of surgery, he emphasized that Bill's chances for survival were still very slim. "You might survive the surgery," Susan remembers the surgeon saying, "but with your immune system so compromised, it's not likely you'd survive the recovery."

Plans were put in place for the surgery anyway, since it seemed to be the only hope. Bill was moved to the surgical floor on the third day. Bill and Susan's spirits were about as low as you could imagine. After all, he'd been given what almost amounted to a death sentence.

At this point, a new doctor entered the story. Susan described him as an angel, claiming he was a lot like the Cary Grant character Dudley, an angel in the movie *The Bishop's Wife*. He told Bill that he would be taking over his case.

This new doctor was very supportive and comforting, pointing out calmly that since there was little chance of Bill surviving the surgery, it would be a better solution to sterilize the lung. He persuaded the surgeon and the infectious disease doctor that this was the best course of action, and on the fourth day the sterilization plans were made. Bill was discharged the next day, to either die or survive, but he was instructed to stay on an array of strong antibiotics until the infection cleared.

Bill survived. In March, five months after the sterilization, the doctor said Bill could "try" to go off the antibiotics. At the onset, infection markers in Bill's case were off the charts and eventually moved down into the 200 range; 20 is the normal range for a healthy person. The doctor told Bill and Susan that, even under the best scenario, Bill would probably never get down to the 30's.

Nevertheless, there was continued improvement, to 120, then 90, then 80 ... but then back to 97. Bill had lost

35 pounds, and he'd been a slim person to start with. He and Susan were devastated until a reading of 68, down from 87, cheered them. Bill had gained some weight, returned to work, and was scheduled for a follow-up appointment in three months unless the development of fever prompted an earlier visit.

This was a reprieve, but there was a problem with the strength and side effects of the drugs (quinolones) Bill was taking; long-term use of quinolones can be debilitating. Bill was anxious to get off them, which he did. However, several weeks later symptoms of coughing and fever returned. Another setback. And so the antibiotic CIPRO was administered for two weeks. Three weeks after he stopped taking the antibiotics, coughing developed. Although Bill was getting pure food and supplements, he was coughing more, became pale and developed a fever. Susan identified a repeating pattern; it seemed like things were going in reverse. She knew that even the thought of needing another round of CIPRO would be a devastating blow for Bill.

Then Susan heard about Precious Waters™ from a friend. She had a very strong hunch it might help. Bill was at the end of his rope and refused to try anything new, but Susan was so convinced that it would help, she ordered three bottles. In May, she started putting a teaspoon in his morning coffee and evening water without his knowing it. Seeing improvement, she increased the dosage to a tablespoon, several times a day.

Bill started to feel better, so on the ninth day, she told him about the nanosilver. They agreed he should keep taking it, despite the fact that Bill was experiencing some diarrhea, cramps and gas pains. A noted oncologist said that these effects were probably not due to any side effect of nanosilver. He explained that those symptoms occur frequently as a result of antibiotic use. Apparently, the antibiotics remove helpful bacteria, thus allowing pathogenic bacteria to overgrow the gut and cause the symptoms. Nevertheless, since these side effects did not subside after an additional two weeks, Bill decided to go off the "silver water." The increase in coughing returned almost instantly so Susan ordered 10 more bottles of Precious Waters™ and convinced him to take a reduced amount of 1 teaspoon a day.

Within two days of starting that regimen, the coughing stopped and there was no more fever. She then increased the amount to 2 teaspoons 2 times a day. Bill stopped taking everything else, including raw food shakes and veggies. There were no more side effects, indicating that the oncologist was likely correct that they'd been caused by the antibiotics.

So what's the conclusion? Well, in late June 2014 Bill underwent new chest X-rays and bloodwork. Bill and Susan got the results that week from a smiling doctor. The infection blood marker count, which was not supposed to reach the 30's, was an amazing 33!

As for the X-rays, they showed that the formerly pus-filled Bullae bubble *no longer appeared to be infected.* And where originally it appeared that the disease had also spread to the healthy right lung? That lung now looked 100% healthy. All indications were that the damaged left lung had improved so much, Bill did not need to come back for another checkup for six months.

Might someone with a different type of lung disease infer from this story that they might experience improvement also? That's up to each individual. Remember, no claims are made for Precious Waters™. According to FDA rules, it is allowed to be sold as a dietary supplement only.

That said, if a disease is caused by a pathogen, virus, bacteria or fungus, we do have the results of laboratory tests mentioned earlier that nanosilver is non-toxic and will effectively kill harmful pathogens. We also have test results from decades ago by Robert O. Becker, M.D., pioneering researcher, surgeon and author. He determined that silver ions were the only metal-based ions that killed pathogens at certain voltage levels, while not harming healthy tissue.

We have other events cited in this book: the results of clinical trials in Kenya; the recent medical experiments showing that silver can make antibiotics many times more effective; and all the anecdotes that follow.

## Chapter 3: Chronic Leukemia, Precious Waters™ & Chemo

Dave, one of Harry's oldest and most trusted friends, flew on his crew into Vietnam. Today, Dave holds a leadership position among a group of retired Continental Airlines pilots. He has a son in Houston who was originally diagnosed with TB in December 2013. In his mid-30s, the son was fatigued, had trouble sleeping, and was experiencing night sweats. A doctor diagnosed him as having chronic leukemia, which is not as fast-growing or dangerous as acute leukemia, but it is a cancer nonetheless.

He was treated at M.D. Anderson, a leading cancer hospital in Houston, with very low-dose chemo, but at the same time he started taking one ounce of Precious Waters™ three times a day, plus baking soda two times a day for about a month, before gradually reducing the amount. Where his white cell count had been between 400,000 and 500,000 when he started, it was in the normal range of 10,000 to 12,000 after five weeks. And where cancer had been found in his bone marrow before, there was no sign of cancer there after the five-week period.

The doctor in charge, who did not know his patient was taking Precious Waters™, was quite pleased. In answer to Dave's question as to how the son's recovery compared to most cases, the doctor replied that while not unprecedented, it could be characterized as "fairly unexpected" on the positive side. Dave's son is now living a normal life, working, sleeping better and feeling much more energetic.

So did the nanosilver help? Dave is absolutely convinced it played a major role, but because chemo was given at the same time, no one can be sure for certain. That's okay, though. The important thing for Dave is that his son is now healthy, and while he is convinced that Precious Waters™ helped significantly, no claims are made.

Unfortunately, Dave also had another story to relate, a sad one about his daughter, a triathlon participant who worked out regularly. She held a degree relating to diet and nutrition, giving her above average knowledge of how to stay healthy. Unfortunately, she developed breast cancer that went undiagnosed for years. It had spread to a Stage 4 cancer and was in her spinal fluid and other places in her body when she started treatment at M.D. Anderson.

Naturally Dave wanted her to take Precious Waters™ along with the chemo, and she did so. To Dave's delight, her counts immediately began improving and she regained a good deal of strength. However, when she advised her doctors that she was taking nanosilver, they told her to stop taking it so they could more accurately measure the effects of the chemo. They meant well, of course, and may not have known much if anything about nanosilver and the science behind it.

Being a conscientious patient with tremendous respect for the doctors at M. D. Anderson and all that they had achieved in battling cancer, she followed their advice. Unfortunately, she died nine months later.

Who knows what would have happened if she had continued to take Precious Waters™ along with the chemo? She still might have died, though Dave feels otherwise. Dave was kind to share this information with me, even though it was troubling for him to speak about it. He hopes that by sharing the story, he might help someone who is unsure about trying Precious Waters™ or using it while undergoing chemo.

The case of Dave's daughter does relate to a common situation in which many people are afraid to take Precious Waters™ either because doctors discourage it or they see something on the internet with negative implications.

## Chapter 4: Fever Blisters & Actinic Keratosis Disappear, Hepatitis C Treatment Assisted

Fever blisters, also known as cold sores and oral herpes, are caused by the herpes simplex virus. They are very contagious and can commonly be transmitted from one person to another simply by kissing. A California man in his sixties had been bothered by fever blisters for some time. The blisters were not only physically painful but also socially embarrassing. While the sores usually heal in two or three weeks, the virus remains, so they can recur regularly.

This man started taking Precious Waters™ in early 2014, and after two months his fever blisters disappeared. He has had no episodes or recurrences since then. More significantly, he had been bothered for a long time by skin rashes on his arms, head and face (some related to previous skin cancers) and all of these have either diminished dramatically or disappeared. As a preventive, both he and his wife take a teaspoon of nanosilver once a day, though he isn't sure they need to.

In another case a 70-year-old Vietnam vet who was exposed to Agent Orange had severe actinic keratosis on his arms. His skin was scaly, rough and fire-engine red according to his wife, a Registered Nurse. The man had bleeding blisters, a common form of pre-cancer, and his wife did not want him to use fluorouracil cream, the most common treatment, because she believed it also destroys healthy cells.

She started spraying her husband's arms twice a day with Precious Waters™ Topical Spray Gel, which is specially formulated to penetrate the skin. At the start, she didn't think it would help much. To her surprise, the raised bumps symptomatic of actinic keratosis nearly disappeared. After using three bottles of the topical spray gel over three weeks, his right arm looked almost normal. His left arm was not as good because it got more sun exposure from driving, but it also improved dramatically.

As an aside, his younger brother, also exposed to Agent Orange in Vietnam, had the same condition, but not as severe. Still, the skin was itchy, inflamed and rough. He applied the gel spray one evening, and the next day he claimed his skin was as smooth as a baby's. He couldn't believe it and immediately bought three more bottles. Another happy coincidence.

### A Few More Anecdotes – Infection, Hepatitis C, Advanced Prostate Cancer

Here are a few more anecdotes about people who took Precious Waters™, in one case as a supplement to conventional therapy. No claims made, no cause-and-effect, but interesting stories nevertheless.

Harry's daughter Theresa had an **undiagnosed infection in her right elbow** that was quite painful, felt hot, and was growing fast. She started taking the Precious Waters™ and in just four days it was gone.

Joanne in North Dakota **had diagnosed Stage 4 Hepatitis C.** She had 15-month-long treatment with conventional drug therapy and showed improvement. Before resuming further treatment with a new, more effective drug that could be administered in 90 days, she took Precious Waters™ aggressively—10 bottles in 38 days.

She said this kept her viral count low, and she believes it assisted in making the second round of conventional therapy so effective. She is now in remission, with no viral load, and intends to take the "silver water" as a preventive, figuring it does no harm and would not prevent detection of the Hepatitis C virus in the event it did return. Her experience gives hope that Precious Waters™ might one day be approved as part of the treatment for Hepatitis C, in combination with drugs.

A 67-year-old fellow in Illinois, Richard H, had **advanced prostate cancer** and was sent home to die in 2008. The doctors expected him to live for only about a week. In April he started taking the nanosilver and continued for a few months. He talked with Harry around Christmas of that year, having just returned from his full-time job on a construction project.

## Chapter 5: Merkel Cell Carcinoma vs Precious Waters™ ... and the winner is....

We don't want to claim that Precious Waters™ has anything to do with fighting, treating or curing any disease, but as noted in the title of this chapter, we can say that Merkel Cell Carcinoma lost by a knockout in the following anecdote.

Harry got very good news one evening in April 2014. Paul, the leader of a Bible study group at his church, is a friend who Harry considers to be an outstanding scholar, as well as a warm and encouraging person. At age 70, he was diagnosed with Merkel Cell Carcinoma, a rare skin cancer that is often considered more deadly than melanoma. Extensive information on the cancer is available at the NIH / National Cancer Institute website:

http://www.cancer.gov/cancertopics/pdq/treatment/merkel cell/Patient/page4

Suggested treatments include surgery, chemotherapy, and radiation. In this man's case, the visible evidence of the cancer was a growth below the nose the size of a peanut shell, pink to grayish purple in color. The surgeon said he would have to remove his upper lip, part of his nose, part of his jaw, surrounding facial tissue, and some lymph nodes, but that with artistic rebuilding with pigskin, he'd look fine. Chemo and radiation would also be part of the treatment after the surgery.

At age 70, Paul figured he'd rather not go through all that, and knowing of Precious Waters™, he decided to try it. He and Harry agreed he should use both the topical spray gel externally and the Precious Waters™ internally. What happened?

Well, no one can say it was due to the nanosilver, but once again, another coincidence. In the same month that he took it, Paul went back to the oncologist who had biopsied and diagnosed him. **The oncologist could find no trace of the carcinoma!**

As noted on the NIH website, this kind of sudden recovery rarely happens, especially not in just a month. Another happy coincidence, nothing more. But Harry and the entire church are very happy that Paul will likely be around for quite some time, and they're very happy he decided to try the nanosilver.

You have to wonder if people with the more common condition of melanoma might enjoy the same happy coincidence if they tried Precious Waters™ and the topical spray gel. It would be nice, even if no cause/effect relationship exists, even if it's due to a simple placebo effect. Harry's goal of helping as many people as possible would be furthered regardless.

Paul volunteered a written testimonial, and he's happy to have his name attached. Harry has the original signed copy, but here are excerpts from his statement:

April 12, 2014

TESTIMONY CONCERNING PRECIOUS WATERS:

My name is Paul Marks. I am 71 years old and was diagnosed with Merkel Cell Carcinoma in January of this year. I discovered a cyst on my upper lip which was biopsied for the diagnosis of Merkel Cell Carcinoma.

I have a weak heart and weak lungs. For those reasons, I decided against the surgery and radiation treatments that were recommended by the doctors.

Through a friend I was aware of Precious Waters and of the success some had as a treatment for cancer. I have been taking the nano silver (Precious Waters) for over two months.

On April 8th I saw an Oncologist .... He looked closely at my lip and stated, "There is no malignancy on your lip." The Merkel Cell cyst was gone after two months of taking Precious Waters. I can only conclude that this resulted from a miracle by God or the Precious Waters…or both.

This is my testimony.

-Paul Marks

That's a simple, straightforward statement, but please remember these are his words only. Although Paul mentioned "treatment for cancer," Harry never makes any claims about Precious Waters and the FDA specifically prohibits any claim that it is a treatment or cure for any disease. However, Paul's testimony should be interesting to anyone with melanoma or aggressive skin cancer, or any other type of cancer, especially if they can't or won't take conventional chemo and radiation treatment.

# Chapter 6:  From Breast Cancer to Gum Disease:  20 Old Testimonials

In April 2014 Harry Watson's wife Donna typed up some old testimonials from people who had used Precious Waters™ or the topical spray gel for a variety of illnesses: shingles; gum and tooth infections; candida; psoriasis; Crohn's Disease; wound healing; sinus infections, and more. The testimonials are reprinted here as Donna keyboarded them, with initials instead of last names to protect privacy. The originals are available to view for anyone who wants to contact Harry.

- I ordered one bottle of Precious Waters on March 6, 2010. I was willing to try anything to help alleviate the stress from **Candida.** I have had this disease for four and one-half years and have tried every known remedy with no success. I now feel the best I have felt in more than four years. I am shocked and pleasantly surprised as to the speed with which Precious Waters reacted to my affliction. I thank you from the bottom of my heart. **John W. – Chicago**
- I have had recurring bouts of **shingles** for years. I've tried all kinds of treatments with no real

effective solution. After applying Precious Waters Spray Gel topically and taking Precious Waters orally, I am now free of any symptoms, including pain and itching after the second application. **Vivian B. – Portland, OR**

- I have had **psoriasis** for as long as I can remember. I am now free of any symptoms after using Precious Waters for three weeks. Keep up the good work. **Jay R. – Arizona**

- Dear Mr. Watson, thank you for introducing me to Precious Waters. I have had **ringworm and skin infections** ever since I left Viet Nam many years ago. My skin is now clear, and I owe it all to you. **Dhac T. – Little Saigon**

- I was diagnosed with **breast cancer** in January, 2010. I didn't start taking Precious Waters until the middle of February. My cancer symptoms have disappeared. **Rhonda D. – Utah**

- Dear Mr. Watson, I have tried many solutions for my **prostate cancer.** None of them appeared to work until I started taking Precious Waters. After six weeks my symptoms have been mitigated, and my blood tests show a reduction in the various test measurements. My doctor is very pleased with my progress, and we are no longer considering surgery. **Rich M. – Fullerton, CA**

- I was diagnosed with **Crohn's Disease** in early 2008. All my symptoms disappeared after two weeks of using Precious Waters. I since have been treated with the Precious Waters™ Spray Gel for second and third-degree burns with amazing results. I will keep both the oral and the topical Precious Waters on hand the rest of my life. **Tara C. – San Diego**

- I am 59 now, and 40 years ago I had a serious road accident which left me with a **scar** at the side of my mouth. This scar caused me great concern for very many years. However, to cut a long story short, I had plastic surgery on two occasions, and this did little or nothing to remove the scar. In fact, on the first occasion it made things worse. Over the years I have tried many types of treatments which have offered no success. Then I ordered the Precious Waters silver solution. I thought, why not put some of this solution on my scar? After all, I have tried nearly everything else! All I can say is that the results are utterly astounding! Here before my eyes, after 40 years, the scar is healing! Fantastic! What more can I say?! This product has got to be the best! **David B**

- This may be hard to believe, but the Precious Waters solution helped save our **Cocker Spaniel's** life. Diagnosed with a severe **liver disease** common to this breed, we were told the dog needed $3,000.00 in transfusions immediately and probably would not survive anyway. We brought him home to rest and go in peace with us. That was one month ago today! Even though the veterinarians cannot explain it, we can. We gave our dog 2 tablespoons of Precious Waters with each meal, three times a day. He's our little Easter Miracle! Thank you! **Kris V**

- I had the opportunity to consult with a client regarding a **non-healing wound to her left leg.** The wound developed in January and had become much worse by March. The client had been receiving professional treatment from a wound care center here in Florida. A variety of solutions, creams, and salves were being used to heal the area, only making the situation worse. I decided to use Precious Waters on the area, and I am pleased to report that after two weeks the wound is closing with a scab. I am really glad I could help, and the client is very pleased with the results. **Karen B**

- Wow, I can't believe it! I had a terrible **sinus headache** which I usually get this time of the year, and it turns into a **sinus infection.** Well, I had this for four days, and I inhaled Precious Waters Spray Gel this morning and, within one half hour the terrible headache was gone and has not returned all day. My sinus has cleared and I can breathe again! All I can say is that Precious Waters is worth its weight in GOLD! In my experience, not even antibiotics have worked this fast. I will never be without Precious Waters in my home! Thanks! **Susan C**

- I had been having some **discomfort in a tooth/gum** area for about a month. I went to the dentist and was told I had an **inflamed periodontal pocket.** My dentist recommended an

antibiotic injection into the pocket, but he was only 50% sure that it would help. It would not be covered by my insurance, and it would cost $138.00. I decided not to have it and just wait and see if it got better or worse on its own. When I got home I was reading about the Precious Waters' silver solution and its bacteria killing effectiveness, so I thought I would try it on my tooth/gum area. Not having a syringe, I took a drink stirrer similar to a little straw. I put it in the bottle, put my finger over one end, lay down and let it drip out around my tooth. In just a couple of hours it was better! It hasn't hurt once since then! Now, when I take it I just swish it around my mouth before I swallow it. I was quite impressed and am spreading the word to all who will listen.
**John H**

▪ Nobody could have been more skeptical of Precious Waters than me. I've tried hundreds of 'health' products that didn't live up to their claims. It was with these past experiences in mind I once again "experimented." A nasty *'something'* was giving me a **raspy throat, headache, pain in the eyes and aches in general** after having felt fine only hours before. My roommate was already miserably ill. I remembered the stories about Precious Waters, and I had an unopened bottle, so I took a teaspoon. Within four hours I was fine. Just to play it safe, I took another teaspoon the following day. The next day I didn't, and I started to get the same symptoms. I took a teaspoon immediately and felt better shortly. I continued taking it for another four days. I've never experienced anything like this. I was amazed. It worked! Not long after that I had the experience of doctoring **a pigeon with a bad wound.** The pigeon got well drinking a teaspoon of Precious Waters added to its daily water. Then, a few days after releasing the pigeon, one of my cockatiels got sick. It was after the pet store closed, and birds often die quickly. I tried the Precious Waters in the bird's drinking water, and it came around fast. I kept it on the product a week as I do with antibiotics. I'll keep Precious Waters on hand from now on. **Mary D**

- I just want to say that I'm getting more enthused about Precious Waters each month! I am exposed to every 'bug' from two school districts here in PA, and every winter spend 5-10 days 'downtime' with some variation of **the flu**. For as long as I can remember—usually during January—I come down with something nasty. However, I've been taking Precious Waters since October, and while everyone in my family and most of our friends have been ill this winter, I have not even had a cold! I'm one of the world's foremost skeptics, I'll confess, but as the winter draws to a close and I continue to feel great, I'm becoming a true believer in this stuff. The testing on Anthrax is another exciting aspect of Precious Waters in

26

these perilous times, as well. Thanks very much, and God bless you! **Dave H – PA**

- I want to share with you my experience with Precious Waters. I was being treated for an **upper respiratory infection** and didn't seem to be getting any better. I had been back to the doctor twice and had my medicine changed both times. I started reading about Precious Waters and decided to give it a try. After taking just one dose of the product I felt a whole lot better. I took another dose before going to bed that night, and when I woke up the next morning I literally jumped out of bed and found that I was feeling better than I had in a long time. I can't say enough about how good this product is! **Penny U**

- My name is Michael W. I recently had a **tooth ache** and, since nothing worked short of pulling out all my teeth, I decided to use Precious Waters on my bad tooth. Not only did it stop the pain, but it also took away the infection that was caused from the bad tooth. My dentist would have given me a prescription to take away the infection, but since I used Precious Waters I didn't need anything else. **Michael W**

- One night I had a really bad **stomach pain** that was just hurting really bad. I felt like my insides were twisting up really bad. I went to bed restless with the pain still there every time I took a breath. When I got up in the morning feeling really frustrated, I remembered that I had a bottle of

Precious Waters. I took only one tablespoon full of the product, and ten minutes later my pain was GONE! Coincidence? I don't think so! I totally believe in Precious Waters! **Nhut H. L**

- I was rather surprised when, after only using Precious Waters for two weeks, my teeth didn't ache anymore. Since a young child I have had major problems with my gums and teeth. **Periodontal pockets and bleeding gums** were problems I had to deal with for literally years and years. I am ecstatic to say my teeth are no longer sensitive to cold or hot. They no longer bleed when I brush them, and my gums are strong and healthy. In fact, my dentist couldn't believe how great they looked. I had to go in for checkups and cleaning every three months. This last time, my dentist gave me a clean bill of health and told me to come back in six months. He said to just keep doing whatever I was doing which is, of course, taking one-half or one teaspoon of Precious Waters. Thank you, Precious Waters, for providing a pure quality product. **Carol L.**

- I wanted to personally let you know about my experience with Precious Waters' silver solution. I was burning a brush pile early in the morning of September 20, 2001. Although I was over 30 feet from the brush pile, some gasoline fumes ignited and severely **burned both my legs.** I immediately went into shock. I put ice on the burns, but incredible pain kept coming back. I then sprayed the Spray Gel on the burns, and immediately the pain went away. Although my legs were numb, I continued to spray the solution on the burns every 15 minutes most of that day. Now, four months later, my legs are almost completely healed. I initially thought I would have extensive scarring and possibly need a skin graft. Now, the scars are barely visible. I have your product to thank for that! **David N**

▪ This is a rather long letter about a very sick dog and your miraculous product. I am writing because I am convinced the nanosilver is keeping my dog alive and healthy. Boudreaux (Boo) is a 10-year-old **English Springer Spaniel.** Boo contracted a "mysterious" liver ailment in January. He underwent a biopsy and was treated with antibiotics. The biopsy showed **severe liver destruction**; however, he seemed to mend and we thought he would be alright. By November he showed further signs of illness. For the next few months we treated him with antibiotics, but there was no improvement. The vets then stopped the antibiotics, fearing he would develop immunity. They said nothing further could be done. Either he would have another biopsy and possibly be treated with steroids, or we would do nothing and eventually his liver would fail.

During the next few months I agonized over what to do. While we did nothing, Boo's greatest danger was developing **secondary bacterial infections** because of his depressed immune system. It was during this period that I frantically searched the web and every place else, looking for something to try and protect him from this danger. That's when a friend at work suggested nanosilver. I did as much research as I could to determine if it was safe for him. The vets were NO help in answering my questions or providing any support for any type of "alternative treatment." In fact, they blew me off...but, having nothing to lose, I started giving it to Boo in November.

In January I took Boo back to Tech. The head vet saw him this time, took one look at Boo and said he looked great. He thought by looking at Boo's overall health that we were probably dealing with a slow infection and could treat and stop the infection, and Boo could probably live on his reduced liver function for many years. The vets did do a biopsy to confirm their diagnosis.

I'll never forget the afternoon they called me after the biopsy. He was absolutely floored. The biopsy revealed that Boo had less than 20% liver function, and by all rights Boo should have been on his death bed. The vet had never seen a liver as damaged and a dog as healthy looking as Boo. He said his system should have been full of bacteria, but there was not a sign of bacteria anywhere. He couldn't believe it. However, his diagnosis was there was nothing we could do to prolong his life. We'd give him steroids to make him feel better, but that my dog would be dead in a matter of months, probably from internal bacterial infections (like e. coli). I again tried to tell him about nanosilver, and his answer was, "yeah, sure."

Well, guess what, it's been 8 months and Boo's still with us. Oh, he has slowed down very much and doesn't feel too good some days. But to look at him you would never know about his liver condition. He has not had one single bacterial problem. Every 80 days I check in with the vets and each time they are expecting me to tell them Boo has died. Well…not yet!

In my mind there is NO DOUBT Boo is alive and healthy today because nanosilver has kept him bacteria free. In fact, it was my 'doubting Dave husband' that gave it the name "Miracle Medicine." Oh, I know it will not cure him, but each month that he remains bacteria free is one more month I have him with me. **Deborah B**

## Chapter 7: Can Precious Waters™ Beat Shingles Pain? The End of Endometriosis?

Here is a story is about a woman with shingles who experienced a happy coincidence when she took Precious Waters™. A few years back this woman, suffering terrible pain from shingles, attended one of Harry Watson's lectures in the Portland OR area. A thin woman, she had suffered terrible pain around her middle and had often been bedridden during the previous 12 years. No treatment seemed to help.

In desperation she used the topical spray gel as well as the Precious Waters™. She let Harry know that she had taken only two ounces of it and had applied the spray gel for only two days, when her pain was suddenly gone.

Harry lost contact with her, so we do not know what happened over the long term, but he does know she got relief from the pain in just two days. This is just one anecdote, and the only one we have for shingles to date.

As for endometriosis, it is interesting to hear stories where people report improvement after using Precious Waters™. Until Harry Watson called one morning in March 2014, I didn't know what endometriosis was. It affects five million women and has no cure, only treatments. For severe, long lasting cases, one of the recommended procedures is major abdominal surgery. Here is a description taken from a women's medical website:

Endometriosis is a common health problem in women. It gets its name from the word "endometrium" (en-doh-MEE-tree-um), the tissue that lines the uterus or womb. Endometriosis occurs when this tissue grows outside of the uterus on other organs or structures in the body. Most often, endometriosis is found on the:

- Ovaries
- Fallopian tubes
- Tissues that hold the uterus in place
- Outer surface of the uterus
- Lining of the pelvic cavity

Other sites for growths can include the vagina, cervix, vulva, bowel, bladder, or rectum. In rare cases, endometriosis has been found in other parts of the body, such as the lungs, brain, and skin. (End of description from website)

So why did Harry call me? Because a woman in McKees Rocks, PA, about five miles northwest of Pittsburgh on the Ohio River, heard about Harry and ordered 10 bottles of Precious Waters™ at the end of December 2013. She ordered it because her daughter, 24, had been suffering severe pain from endometriosis for ten years, virtually her entire adult life. She had been under medical treatment but nothing had helped significantly.

The daughter had wanted to join a military service,

but she was rejected because of the endometriosis and its attendant severe pain. She had tried attending college, but the pain overwhelmed her. The woman wanted her daughter to try Precious Waters™ to see if it might help.

Harry didn't know any of this history until he heard from her again three months later. She emailed Harry, wanted to order five more bottles, and added "God bless you." Harry called her to let her know there was a price break at six bottles, so a sixth bottle wouldn't cost her much more. He then inquired as to why she was ordering more and she told him the story of her daughter's progress so far.

In early January 2014, the daughter started taking two teaspoons of the nanosilver morning, noon and night. *By coincidence or something else, the daughter's pain lessened almost right away and soon stopped. Not only that, but there were no longer signs of any tumors on any of her female organs.*

The reason the woman was ordering more was because her daughter had been accepted for military service and was reporting the next day. The woman was very concerned that the endometriosis pain might return, so she wanted to be sure her daughter had a supply while in the service.

The doctors who had been treating the daughter for almost 10 years were dumbfounded because there is no known cure for endometriosis. The woman did not tell them about her daughter taking the nanosilver because she expected their reaction would be negative.

Harry was of course overjoyed to hear of the

daughter's improvement. Success stories are why he started the company in his late eighties — to help as many people as possible experience these coincidences with affordable, high quality nanosilver. He originally thought only of patients with cancer because he attributed his seemingly miraculous cure to the nanosilver, but he has since learned that silver has a long history of fighting infections, and some believe it can positively affect any disease caused by a virus, bacteria or fungus.

Again, no claims are made, but to hear that taking this unique form of nanosilver and recovering from a disease that affects 5 million women coincidentally happened at the same time, is heartening indeed. Whatever the cause for her improvement, the daughter has her life going in the direction she wants, free of pain at long last.

# Chapter 8: Toothache, Blood in the Urine & Stage 4 Prostate Cancer

In February 2014 a woman ordered some Precious Waters™ from Harry Watson in hopes it would help her with a toothache she'd developed after an injection at the dentist six months earlier.

Good news. The toothache is gone! Even better news? Blood in her urine—a condition she'd suffered from for years—disappeared after a few weeks of taking the nanosilver daily. She'd tried a number of cures previously, including various antibiotics, but to no avail. A respected California physician who'd treated her for years without success, was so impressed by her improvement that he ordered 20 bottles for other patients.

Apparently he was impressed enough with what he saw in his other patients that he inquired with Harry about buying it in quantities large enough to sell under his own private label.

This physician is an M.D., a Fellow of the American College of Physicians (FACP), a national organization of internal medicine physicians, and a Fellow of the American College of Allergy, Asthma & Immunology (FACAAI). He has a large and loyal following of over 800 patients.

**Stage 4 Prostate Cancer**

Here's a question. Might Precious Waters™ help beat Stage 4 prostate cancer? Certainly no such claim can be made. However, you might be interested in another coincidence. In November 2013, Harry Watson sent it to a fellow named Jerry who had been diagnosed with Stage 4 prostate cancer. Harry suggested he take it along with a daily dose of baking soda to help make his system less acidic. Jerry did NOT show any improvement in November, December or January. He and his wife Margaret were losing hope, ready to give up. Harry encouraged them to persist, telling them that Stage 4 cancer can't be expected to quickly recede.

They continued. The doctor kept changing Jerry's chemo "cocktail" in his efforts to find the most effective treatment, but the nanosilver and baking soda were a constant. Things finally changed dramatically for the better. Jerry's CEA marker for cancer went from 18.3 on February 10, 2014, to 6.7 on March 10, 2014... *with no chemo treatments during that time because his white cell count was too low.* Today, he's feeling much better.

Margaret emailed Harry: "The 6.7 shocked the doctor and he came back to the infusion room to talk with Jerry personally and tell him this was a shock to him and he had to give him the good news!"

Instead of chemo again in two weeks, the doctor wanted to wait three weeks. As Margaret shared with Harry: "When we told him about the Precious Waters and the baking soda, he just shook his head and told Jerry, 'Well, if you think the nanosilver and baking soda is doing this, then keep it up,'... but naturally he had to give the chemo drugs the credit."

As a matter of fact, Harry doesn't care who or what gets the credit, as long as Jerry recovers and lives a life he feels good about. Jerry and Margaret give the credit to the "Great Physician Upstairs" and to the Precious Waters™ and they are especially happy that Jerry is not even sick from the chemo. Margaret thanked Harry for his encouragement and for talking with her, but it is Harry who is thankful to see another person feeling better and seemingly beating cancer … and as noted, he doesn't care who gets the credit.

# Chapter 9: Totally Paralyzed Minister Speaks and Moves Eyes

Talk about interesting anecdotes! This story involves a condition that has never before been associated with Precious Waters™ … even by coincidence.

About three years ago a pastor in a southern California church fell ill after preaching a Sunday morning sermon. He developed severe pain in his stomach during the day so his wife took him to the ER in the local hospital that evening. They performed a few tests but no diagnosis was made.

He was sent home but continued to get worse. When he returned to the ER the next day, they discovered a blood clot near his liver, which blocked the flow to his intestines. Doctors operated and removed a lot of his intestines, and later he also underwent brain surgery.

Eventually he became totally paralyzed, and could not speak or even move his eyes. Seeing the severity of his condition, the church elders arranged for him and his family to be sent to Chicago, where he could get treated by top doctors. After some months there, it became apparent there was nothing those doctors could do to improve his condition, so the family returned to California with the pastor, who needed continuing close care. Church members volunteered to become involved in his daily care.

One of them knew about Precious Waters™ and suggested there would be no harm in his trying it, on the slight chance that it would make him less vulnerable to opportunistic viruses that could ultimately make a ferocious onslaught to his immune system. It was provided to him at no cost.

The pastor was supposed to take baking soda with the nanosilver, but his paralysis made it difficult to swallow the baking soda; he was able to ingest only a little bit of it. For the most part, the only change in his care regimen was that he started taking nanosilver regularly, with a little baking soda.

For a month there was no visible change in his condition, but the hope was that the nanosilver was in some way assisting his immune system to fight off viruses. At that time, there wasn't much expectation that he would show any visible improvement.

That all changed on a Sunday shortly afterward, when a man at the church turned to the pastor and wished him good morning. He was quite surprised when he heard an extremely weak whisper in reply, "Good morning Michael." In the weeks that followed, church members noted that the pastor's eyes no longer drooped so much, and he could actually move his eyes around in different directions.

Within a few months he was able to also type out messages on a keyboard. These weren't just any messages. They were brief, uplifting messages to members of the church.

Imagine the difference it made for an intelligent, compassionate person to go from being unable to communicate in any way at all, to authoring these helpful messages. That kind of elation was personally and emotionally shared by Jill Bolte Taylor in her book, *My Stroke of Insight.* The pastor hasn't written a book yet, but life for him has got to be a whole lot richer and more rewarding, regardless of how much further he progresses.

This is just an anecdote with absolutely no scientific significance, **and there is no logical way to conclude that his improvements were in any way connected to taking nanosilver.** It's quite possible he would have improved on his own, without ever taking nanosilver. At best, perhaps it helped his immune system in some way.

Still, it is curious that someone who had been totally paralyzed for nearly three years started to speak, move his eyes and type out messages… just a little over six weeks after he started to take Precious Waters™. No one can or should claim cause and effect, but we can all be happy about this remarkable coincidence.

# Chapter 10: Stomach Cancer, Brain Cancer, Warts... All Music to Harry's Ears

It is always music to Harry's ears when someone calls and tells him they are feeling better after taking Precious Waters™. In November 2013 he got a call from a gentleman in Ocala FL, who had been taking it for five weeks. He had a cancer in his stomach that was similar in many ways to Harry's cancer years earlier.

This fellow had recently undergone an operation where the doctors removed a large tumor from his abdomen and told him he had a maximum of one year left to live, with no expectation of recovery. His cancer, like Harry's, had a lot of mucous attached to it and he felt ill at the time he started to take nanosilver. Most of the time he was flat on his back.

At any rate, he called to order more nanosilver and to tell Harry that he was feeling better and making great progress; he was no longer flat on his back as he had been, and had a much brighter outlook. Nothing makes Harry happier than to get this kind of feedback. As always, no cause/effect relationship is claimed.

**But Small Things Can Make Music Too**

Warts certainly are not the reason most people choose to try Precious Waters™, but here are two interesting events.

**Wart Since High School**

A man in his sixties in Peoria IL was taking it orally for other purposes. Since high school he'd had a wart on the top of his head, and it hurt him every time he hit it with a comb. It was the size of a quarter, maybe a bit larger, he said. At any rate, as he continued to take the nanosilver, it disappeared. Wonderful coincidence, even if it was only a wart!

**Donna Sings a Happy Tune About Precious Waters™ Gel Spray**

Harry's wife Donna had two warts. One was on the back of her hand, between the thumb and forefinger. When she took nanosilver internally it stopped growing but did not shrink. When she started to also apply the spray gel, which is specially formulated to penetrate the skin, the wart shrank and sloughed off within 5 days.

The story was the same for another wart on Donna's hip. It was large both horizontally across the skin and vertically above it. When she started to apply the gel spray while also taking Precious Waters™ internally, it disappeared in about a week.

The wart results should not be too surprising. Silver kills infections from bacteria, fungi and viruses, and warts are largely believed to be virus-caused. It stands to reason silver should kill them off, though no claims are made.

**Three More Quick Stories … Music Maestro Please!**
In late September 2013 Harry had three people call him in one week with good news.

A lady in Mexico named Cookie was sent home to die because of her **brain cancer.** A relative decided to make a documentary that the family could keep to remember her. It was supposed to be mainly about her last days and things she might want to say in parting.

At around the same time, Cookie started taking nanosilver and baking soda, and dramatically improved. She still had one tumor, but she began to function each day in ways she couldn't previously. The relative making the documentary was beside himself with joy. He now figures the documentary will be about a remarkable recovery, and he is eager for people to learn about it.

Another call Harry received was from a medical doctor in Ohio who was initially doubtful that Precious Waters™ and baking soda could help his **prostate cancer.** He asked Harry to send him all the technical information available, and then ordered six bottles that were shipped on September 21, 2013.

A little over a week later, the doctor called Harry to exclaim, "This stuff works!" He ordered six more bottles. When Harry asked why he needed more so soon, he replied that he was giving it to some of his patients.

The third story is about a fellow from India, who wanted to do something to help his father with liver cancer. He heard about Precious Waters™, so he purchased ten bottles. He called back during the last week in September to order 20 more bottles, and told Harry his father was much improved.

Again, no claims are made in any of these stories, and nothing is documented. But for Harry, news about even a single person making major strides in beating an illness or infection is cause for great joy. Harry lives for such feedback. It confirms that he is doing what he was meant to do.

## Chapter 11: Cancer & HIV Anecdotes–One Leads to Clinical Study in Kenya

The clinical trials carried out in Kenya were mentioned earlier in this book, but here is the story behind the woman whose HIV started it all. She was HIV-positive and was not permitted by her doctor to get pregnant because of the risk of transmitting the disease to the baby. Long story short, she took a teaspoonful of Precious Waters™ every day for 33 days, and coincidentally got better, no longer testing positive for HIV.

A non-profit holds meetings in Africa on occasion, inviting people who have experienced positive improvements in their condition to attend and relate their experiences. The woman went to one of the meetings, which included a representative of The Gates Foundation, and told them how she had improved. Her story was so impressive that they encouraged more testing, indicating that if further testing proved out, they might consider providing funding for a clinical trial. That funding never developed, but this was part of the impetus behind the Kenyan trials mentioned earlier.

Following is the letter from one of the medical professionals in Kenya who administered Precious Waters™ as one element in the treatment of patients. His original communication contained photos which are not reproduced here. They show a remarkable difference in appearance. The letter was forwarded, which is why there are three names in it. The woman referenced in the story above is the second woman mentioned in the letter below.

—- **Forwarded Message** —-
**From:** Joseph
**To:** Charles
**Sent:** Thursday, October 6, 2011 8:33 AM
**Subject:** RE: Nanosilver Testimonials
Perry,

Hope you're well. Further to our conversation, I have attached three pictures of the same lady (Alice) who's been using our product after having gone through a severe form of cancer called Acitis of the stomach. The picture bearing two images shows her (Right side picture) was taken before she got sick. The one where she's bald (Left side picture) was taken when I met her in May 2011 while going through Chemotherapy at Upper Hill Medical center (Nairobi Radiotherapy clinic) one of the leading hospitals in town.

This picture to the right was taken right in our offices in town on Tuesday the 4th October 2011.

This is the kind of life changing scenarios we are having with Precious Waters. It's humbling.

The last picture here to the left is of a lady (Lucy) who's been battling HIV/AIDs for over 19 years and she has been on ARV's for over 10 years. Her CD4 count has never been past the 400 mark and **after taking Precious**

Waters NanoSilver for a month, her current CD4 count is 829. She did not have hair for over 3 years and her head was bald as a man's. This is a huge improvement considering that she can now conceive a baby as she's free from the risk of transmitting the disease to her new born child. Her viral load has drastically dropped to barely traceable levels. I will be sending over her previous photos when she didn't have hair for over 3 plus years due to fungal infections.

Regards,

Joseph

Managing Director

**HIV Cure (?) Claim Being Monitored**

Here is an article reporting on the work of the late Dr. Barasa Simon Situma of Kenya. Four people apparently "cured" of HIV were being monitored for several months to see if they remained with no traceable viral load. One of the "agents" mentioned in the last paragraph is Precious Waters™. **Again, no claims are made or implied,** and there were three drugs also administered here, including methotrexate, a well-known and powerful cancer drug. Here is the article:

THE HABARI NETWORK: **Simon Barasa-Situma – a Kenyan researcher reports success in providing HIV cure** (Posted on May 13, 2013 – 1:35 pm)

A Kenyan researcher, Dr. Simon Barasa-Situma of the Technical University of Kenya, has modified the world's first recorded HIV "cure" and says it has worked effectively on four of his patients and that another 18 currently under observation "are doing well."

"Consecutive tests show they carry no virus, but we have to monitor them for at least six to 12 months to be sure they are free of HIV," explained Barasa-Situma, during a presentation at the Second World Virology and Microbiology Conference in New York.

"I have demonstrated the HIV cure in two people by stopping rapid multiplication of CD4 progenitor cells in the bone marrow, where the HIV virus hides to avoid elimination by the immune system and thus achieved the first complete cure without bone marrow transplantation," Barasa-Situma said.

His treatment, he says, is based on the world's first known cure of HIV, that of Timothy Ray Brown, 47, who was diagnosed with HIV in 1995 and put on Antiretroviral drugs, but in 2006 developed leukemia and, for this reason, was given a bone marrow transplant with a rare gene mutation that provides natural resistance to HIV.

"Removing the bone marrow, where the CD4 cells replicate, denied the virus the capacity to replicate and consequently the patient was free of HIV," says Barasa-Situma. Since the new bone marrow was resistant to the virus, the already existing bugs in circulation and from the secondary reservoirs—which include the brain, glands, intestines, and skin—could not create new hideouts, hence the ultimate eradication of the virus.

Bone marrow transplantation is a very expensive, specific, and dangerous procedure, which makes Brown's treatment impossible to apply to the more than 30 million people with HIV. However, according to Barasa-Situma, purging the virus from some specific locations where it seems to hide is the way out.

"This means there is a reservoir in the body where the virus is hiding and where the antiretroviral drugs are not able to reach. The hideout is in some parts of the bone marrow. Get rid of this reservoir and, theoretically, you are home and dry," Barasa-Situma says, adding that he has achieved this using a method that comprises the use of a cancer drug (methotrexate) in combination with other agents. Two patients who have undergone the therapy, he adds, have shown no signs of the virus for the past six months.

# Chapter 12: California Woman is "Walking Miracle" After Brain Tumor

Mary M, an athletic 53-year-old woman in southern California, played tennis regularly and was active continually, as any mother of four boys would be. In April of 2014 she experienced nausea and a headache for three days. She didn't think much of it, but her sister, a Physician's Assistant, became alarmed upon learning of the situation. She insisted that Mary go to local ER immediately and have someone else drive her.

Mary followed her sister's advice. Her son dropped her off, and as luck would have it, there were no patients there at the time, so she was seen immediately. She felt sheepish telling the ER staff that she had come because of something as simple as a headache and nausea, but when she sat down to fill out the forms required, she immediately threw up.

She could still function normally, but the medical staff wanted a thorough checkup, including a CAT scan and MRI. After those tests, a neurosurgeon informed her she had a brain tumor, and they didn't know if it was benign or malignant, so they'd need to operate. This was at 5 p.m. in the evening; they scheduled the surgery for 11 a.m. the next morning.

The surgery was successful. The surgeon removed 100% of the tumor and some of the tissue around the borders. Mary was fully functional soon afterwards. In fact, she recovered quickly and was out of the hospital just three days after the surgery.

The bad news, however, was that the tumor was a glioblastoma (GBM), a primary brain tumor in humans. The oncologist put Mary on a regimen of 30 treatments of radiation and chemotherapy, five days a week for six weeks, with the radiation in the morning and a strong chemo by pill in the evening.

The radiation treatment was particularly challenging. Mary couldn't move while the intense radiation was directed at her brain, so she had to wear a confining mask that was then clamped to the table. The staff were particularly reassuring and encouraging, which helped Mary get through the ordeal.

She was in only the second day of this regimen when, by a happy coincidence, she heard about Harry Watson and Precious Waters™. A close friend of hers was talking with a teacher who told her that, despite being exposed to all the viruses and flu that kids bring to school, she never got sick because she took "silver water." She then mentioned Harry's personal story.

The friend urged Mary to look into it. "I know that when anyone gets cancer," Mary recalls her saying, "all your friends and relatives will start telling you about dozens of remedies including teas, certain foods, herbs and more, but this seems different, so please call the man." Mary went to the website of Precious Waters Inc., and was impressed enough to email Harry. This was on a Saturday and she didn't expect a reply until Monday.

Instead she got a reply almost immediately from Harry telling her to "call me now." Luckily, Mary lived in the same town as a member of Harry's family and Harry had been planning a visit that day. He ended up hand-delivering bottles of nanosilver to Mary so that she could get started on it right away. Mary was happily surprised to find that, as the weeks progressed, she suffered none of the common side effects of strong radiation and chemo. She never got nauseous or fatigued and lost only a little bit of hair. She also didn't develop the sores that often develop during such treatment.

Mary's oncologist, who she considers to be outstanding in many ways, was taken back when Mary asked if she could play tennis. "I don't have too many brain tumor patients asking me if they can play tennis, Mary," she said, "and I don't know what you're doing, but whatever it is, keep it up."

Mary not only played tennis, but also attended an athletic "boot camp" and used a treadmill regularly. While continuing to take an ounce of Precious Waters™ three times a day, Mary also changed her diet to organics, started drinking green tea, got off sugars and white flour, and ate more vegetables and fruits.

After the six week treatment, the doctors waited two weeks before the next MRI. Mary continued with the nanosilver during that time. On July 9, 2014, a date Mary will always remember, some happy doctors informed her she was "totally clear" with no trace of a tumor and the swelling had decreased substantially. Equally impressive, her white blood cell count was in the normal range and her platelets actually increased, which is almost unheard of.

The oncologist then put her on a chemo maintenance regimen of five days of chemo, then 23 days off. That is to continue for some months. When it stops, she will continue taking Precious Waters™ as a preventive, because she knows that hers was an aggressive cancer which historically comes back.

When her primary care physician saw her recently, his mouth fell open. "You're a walking miracle!" he exclaimed. He had followed her case closely and was deeply disturbed when the initial news of the GBM tumor was faxed to him. "People with this tumor wind up in wheelchairs or confined to bed, and many don't make it," he told her, "but here you are with totally normal bloodwork and looking as fit and healthy as anyone could want."

Harry Watson will second that impression, saying that he was totally surprised when, expecting to meet a sickly woman, he met instead someone as full of energy as a bubbly teenager. For her part, Mary had expected to meet "an old man" and was equally surprised to meet a vital, youthful and energetic 92-year-old who seemed years younger.

Mary is thankful for all that has transpired. She said she had "the worst diagnosis but the best outcome," and she attributes it in large part to the Precious Waters™. She gives plenty of credit to all the caring medical professionals who treated her and to the chemo/radiation regimen, but she feels strongly that it was more than just a "coincidence" that her remarkable recovery and lack of debilitating symptoms happened at the same time she took nanosilver regularly.

She is thankful now for each day and insists that she will be able to laugh about it with Harry in ten years, during which time she expects to let a number of people know about Precious Waters™. Harry as always makes no claims.

# Chapter 13: Some Stories From 2014 to 2017

### Illinois Woman in her 70s Beats Lymphoma Cancer Discovered by Accident

Early in 2017 a 74-year-old Illinois woman experienced severe shoulder pain and some underarm pain as well. She was taken to the hospital where a CT scan was conducted for a possible heart problem. The scan showed no heart problem. Instead doctors found three free-floating tumors in her abdomen which they believed were cancerous. It would take a month of tests and preparation before treatment could be started.

I spoke with her daughter in August 2017 and learned this woman's story. In the same discussion the daughter shared with me a "back story" about her father who had remarried and lived in Missouri. The daughter explained that her father had been diagnosed with leiomyosarcoma, a rare soft tissue and bone cancer. After normal treatment had not resulted in any improvement, he had been "sent home to die." The daughter lives in a section of Peoria IL where a lot of people had used Precious Waters™ nanosilver, so she knew about it and recommended that her father start taking some each day.

He followed her advice. The man was 6'3" and weighed only 125 pounds when he was sent home, but had already gained 14 pounds while on the silver for a relatively short time. At that time, however, a specialist agreed to treat the man with his version of conventional treatment, with no promise of improvement or prolonged life. He was willing to treat him, however, only if he stopped taking the nanosilver. Her father chose to have this specialist treat him, stopped taking the nanosilver, and died not too long afterward.

As any reader of my blog or book knows, neither Harry Watson nor I recommend keeping any information from medical professionals, but each person will make his or her own decision in that regard. In this case, with her father's experience still in mind, the daughter told her mother that, during the month they were waiting for treatment, she would start giving her nanosilver daily, but she would not order it unless her mother agreed not to tell the doctors that she was taking it. The daughter knew the doctors would advise her against taking the nanosilver.

The mother agreed to take the nanosilver during that month and during treatment. When treatment was ready to start, the doctors ordered a PET scan to help diagnose the type of cancer and staging, but they could find only the largest of the three tumors that had been previously discovered. The other two had disappeared! But this time they detected a small tumor in her spleen as well. Because it had already spread to another part of the body, they classified her cancer as Stage 4 Double-Hit High Grade Large B-Cell non-Hodgkin's Lymphoma and gave her only a 40% chance of survival at the time they started treatment.

It was a very strenuous treatment, a four-cocktail combination of chemotherapy that they gave her over 5 days in the hospital in a continuous drip, every 3 weeks for 6 treatments. Naturally they expected the normal ravages of chemotherapy would become evident. They were soon to be quite surprised, however, and the oncologist was shocked at how well she was doing during the chemotherapy.

She went on walks almost every day, even when she was in the hospital! She did lose 12 pounds and lost her hair in the early phase of the treatments, but then stabilized and never lost weight after that. In fact she gained two pounds by the end of her treatment, again to the surprise of the doctors.

PET scans taken between July 31st and August 2nd showed no trace of cancer, and although it is generally accepted that no cancer patient is totally free of cancer, which is considered only in "remission," doctors could not find any significant trace of it. So on August 8th, 2017, they considered her "cancer-free."

No claims are ever made that Precious Waters™ nanosilver ever cures anything, and in this case there was extensive chemotherapy and many people were praying for the recovery of this woman. Also, as many clinical tests involving placebos have shown, a person's beliefs can be a big factor in whether, and the extent to which, they recover. Still, the woman's daughter is firmly convinced that nanosilver played a key role in protecting her mother from the harmful effects of chemotherapy. Aside from the many coincidental improvements experienced by several people in her section of Peoria when they took nanosilver, she was also impressed by the fact that two of the tumors in her mother's abdomen had disappeared by the time treatment started.

She is also influenced by her own recent experience. She and her husband's feet and knees have hurt for years, just a pain they have lived with. Her doctor is a functional medicine doctor, and had given her an article claiming that many common conditions are due to the Epstein Barr virus. (The article referred to claims made in the best-selling book *Medical Medium* by Anthony William.) She followed a specific diet and took several supplements along with the silver to try and cure the EBV and possibly a thyroid condition as well.

During the diet, supplements and silver, their pain went away. But after they stopped the diet regimen their feet and knees began to hurt again right away. When they thought about what must have been helping, they decided it might well be the silver. Within 2 days of taking the silver again, the pain was gone in their feet and knees, and hasn't come back. Again, no claims are ever made, but she is convinced the nanosilver helped. She could be wrong of course, but why not enjoy a "happy coincidence?"

## Pennsylvania Man in his Mid-70s Free from Esophageal Cancer – Took Chemo, Radiation and Precious Waters ™ Nanosilver

A 75-year-old Pennsylvania man was diagnosed with esophageal adenocarcinoma cancer and heard about

Precious Waters™ nanosilver before starting chemotherapy and radiation. He started taking the nanosilver and baking soda (to make his system more alkaline) on February 12, 2017, and started four sessions of chemotherapy on February 20th, which lasted through March 31st. He also had 28 radiation treatments.

Fortunately, the adenocarcinoma version of esophageal cancer is easier to treat and in this case was still a tumor in the wall of the esophagus. Nevertheless, the surgeon recommended an operation that would involve fashioning an esophagus out of part of the stomach lining, which carries some significant risks, including infections and the reconstructed lining "falling apart."

The man and his wife decided against the operation, and instead, when the chemo and radiation were complete, opted to have him simply take a small amount of the nanosilver along with baking soda in water every day. When they recently visited their gastroenterologist in May 2017, he remarked that "If you weren't my patient, I wouldn't know where to look for the cancer. There is no sign of it."

The other doctors involved were quite surprised at the rapid improvement and this apparent total remission.

The natural assumption is that the chemotherapy and radiation worked well to eliminate the tumor. That might well be the case. But the man and his wife believe that the nanosilver played a significant part in the remission and the rapid progress he made. It certainly did no harm! That is one reason they chose to stick with nanosilver and avoid the operations and related testing that they feared, correctly or not, might have caused more physical problems.

As for Harry and Donna Watson, no claims are ever made. If it is just a coincidence that this man was taking nanosilver along with the chemo and radiation while he made rapid progress, that is of no concern. They are simply happy to share in the joy of this couple, who intend to have the man continue taking Precious Waters™ nanosilver indefinitely.

**Note:** This man stopped taking nanosilver at some point, figuring he was cured. As of late 2019 the cancer has returned. No cause and effect implied.

## Australian Man Reduces "Forest" of Melanoma to 8 and Counting

On June 23rd, 2016, a man from Australia ordered one bottle of Precious Waters ™ gel spray to start treating what he described as a "forest" of melanoma sores all over his body, especially his legs, back and chest, so thick in many places you could not see the skin. He had tried "everything," he said, but nothing helped. He was scared and shared that his future looked grim. Melanoma after all is a deadly skin cancer that, if not treated, can grow inward and ultimately cause death.

With just the first spraying of the gel spray, it took away all his "wowies," he said, referring to the pain. Over the next four months he ordered 85 bottles of Precious Waters™ nanosilver water and 89 of the gel spray, probably many times more than anyone else has used them for a single condition by a factor of 7 or 8, but he obviously feels it was worth it. His November 3 email to Harry started this way:

**"I'm still beating this malady that wants to win, but it's not going to win! I'm down to 8 little monsters on my back now, this is a real good scene to what it was!"**

Shipping charges to Australia for that many bottles are costly, but this man has never mentioned or complained about the cost. When you consider the alternatives, that's understandable. What's a bright outlook on life and freedom from pain worth? No claims here whatsoever. Just another gratifying example of a coincidence where someone gets great results at the same time they happen to be taking Harry's nanosilver! For Harry, the joy is in hearing from all these people who are so happy to get past challenging physical maladies.

## 2017 Update: Australian Man No Longer Has Lesion Under Tongue – "Massive Improvement to my Lifestyle"

The gentleman from Australia sent the following email to Harry and Donna in January 2017:

"And a great new year to both of you, Donna and Harry. The lesion under my tongue seems to have just gone back to normal skin now… huge relief for sure!! All my other little fellas seem to have near quit…

There are traces of skin activity in places like my knuckles from holding steering wheels all these years!!

This is just a patience exercise… keep at them and

continue treating. They get itchy?!

Pretty warm here at this time of year. Will hop onto my cycle and go downtown for a coffee with friends. Really this is a massive improvement to my lifestyle… well done!!!!

Kindest regards, John"

## Texas Man Beats Aggressive Stomach Cancer

A 69-year-old Texas man had surgery in July 2014 to remove an intestinal cancer in his stomach that had also enflamed his liver. It was followed by chemotherapy. A year later, in July 2015, doctors told him that tests showed, unfortunately, it had come back and was aggressive.

At that time he contacted Harry Watson and started to take Precious Waters™ nanosilver, an ounce 2x a day for a month, then a reduced amount, a teaspoon twice a day, for the months of August, September and October. Then on Monday, November 2nd of 2015, tests showed no sign of the cancer.

There will be a PET scan in two months to determine if the cancer has come back. In the meantime, this man, his very happy wife and two daughters, will be celebrating. And he will continue taking the nanosilver as what he considers a preventive.

As always, Harry Watson is delighted, but makes absolutely no claims. He too is happy that once again a coincidence has occurred — someone taking PW nanosilver and recovering from an infection or disease. The Texas gentleman has promised to get back to Harry to let him know the results of the scan in two months.

## Update on Texas Man With Stomach Cancer and Skin Lesion

The 69-year-old Texas man had a PET scan in January 2016, and it showed no signs of any cancer. Not only that, his appetite and strength have returned, he regularly runs 20 minutes on a treadmill, and he is back to what he considers a healthy 250 pounds after his weight had fallen to 226 pounds. No one can claim that the nanosilver helped, but he feels strongly that it did, and that it contributed to his rapid recovery, so he continues to take a small amount daily.

Part of the reason he believes it helped is that he also had a lesion on his leg that was very sensitive. If he hit his leg on that spot, it started bleeding. It got bad enough so that he had to put a bandage over it. The doctors said it wasn't cancerous but wanted to cut it out. Instead he opted to use only the Precious Waters™ Spray Gel on it, starting in December 2015. Just two months later, in February 2016, he reported that it had healed and closed up, with no more signs of any bleeding even if he rubs it or cleans it vigorously in the shower. He treated it with nothing else, so he gives all the credit to the Spray Gel.

Again, no claims are made. That is only his opinion.

## Montana Man Beats Cancer with Chemo, Also Took Nanosilver

An 80-year-old Montana man living near Great Falls was diagnosed with non-Hodgkins B-Cell Lymphoma in his stomach and started chemo on May 21, 2015. His tumor was originally about the size of a fruit jar lid, 3″ according to his wife Barbara. He had 6 sessions of chemo three weeks apart. In mid-July he also ordered 6 bottles of Precious Waters™ nanosilver from Harry Watson and started taking it daily. On August 31st, his oncologist declared him cancer-free.

This is an interesting man, very healthy his entire life, except for diabetes which he kept under tight control. According to Barbara, he was an unusually determined man, so it was easy for him to keep the diabetes under control. As an example of his determination, she related the story of how he won a 2015 Subaru Legacy with all the bells and whistles by winning a contest. The challenge was to see who could sit in a Subaru the longest, getting out only 10 minutes every 2 hours. He was declared the winner after sitting in it for 17 days!!!! He was also very active his entire life, maintaining a fleet of 109 trucks for the State of Montana.

Now no claims can ever be made for Precious Waters™ nanosilver, but in this case it shows that taking the nanosilver along with chemo did no harm. This man and his wife Barbara, with whom I spoke, both maintain that they "know" the nanosilver played a big part in beating this cancer, and Barbara stated that when he started taking it, his Ph level became much more alkaline and less acidic, which is a positive for anyone fighting cancer. When she ordered more bottles from Harry, she thanked him for doing what he does, and asked him not to stop. It is entirely possible, of course, that the chemo alone got rid of the cancer. But they believe so strongly that the nanosilver helped, they advised a neighbor with a cancer tumor to start taking it, and he has already ordered some.

There was a well-publicized study two years ago that indicated when silver was taken along with an antibiotic, the antibiotic was many times more effective, up to 1000% more effective. It is possible that the nanosilver made the chemo much more effective in this case, but that cannot be proven and no claims are made. It's another happy coincidence though.

### California Woman Beats Colon Cancer

This story was already a few years old when I heard about it in July 2015. A good friend of Harry Watson's has a sister in her 70s, who lives in California. A few years back she was diagnosed with colon cancer, with a tumor in her stomach. Doctors were going to operate to remove the cancer, but first she had to undergo radiation. She had undergone radiation three times, and wasn't tolerating it all that well, so Harry's friend advised his sister to stop the radiation and start taking Precious Waters™ nanosilver.

He ordered 6 bottles from Harry and had it shipped to his sister, who started taking it daily over a period of about four weeks.

She then went back to her doctors to have them remove the tumor, but by that time the tumor had shrunk and the doctors could find no trace of cancer. They were of course puzzled but advised her to keep doing whatever she was doing, because the results were positive.

No claims are made here, of course, but this woman continues to take nanosilver on a regular basis. She also continues an active social life, is a very healthy woman, drives from CA to Las Vegas on occasion, and enjoys the results of the very happy coincidence where the cancerous tumor shrank and became non-cancerous at the same time she happened to start taking the nanosilver.

## California Woman Beats Bladder Infection

On July 20th, 2014, a woman in Huntington Beach, California, called Harry and ordered 10 bottles of Precious Waters™ nanosilver. She said she was suffering from a bladder infection. On July 28th, just 8 days later, she called and ordered 50 more bottles!

With the 2nd order she explained to Harry that the pain and irritation associated with the infection ended within three days when she started taking nanosilver. She then missed a day and it started to come back. She resumed taking it and the symptoms once again subsided.

Harry suggested that she continue to take it for four weeks from the time she started, and that 10 bottles would be enough to last for that period. She wanted the 50 bottles anyway, she explained, because she wanted each of her three daughters to have it on hand, and she wanted a supply on hand for herself. As always, no claims made, just another happy coincidence.

## Has Nanosilver Been Taken By Kids?

It would seem logical that nanosilver would be just as

harmless for kids as it has been for adults. I called Harry Watson to learn if any kids had taken it, and he could recall only one instance where a child had taken it internally.

A neighbor of Harry's in CA a few years back had a beautiful baby girl, 2-1/2 years old, who had salmonella, with its attendant vomiting and diarrhea. She'd had it for more than two days, and whatever the doctors had used to treat it didn't seem to be effective. They knocked on Harry's door and asked if Precious Waters™ nanosilver might help, and Harry gave them some. They spooned just a little bit into her mouth, and the next day she was a lot better.

She later developed pinkeye, and her mother sprayed a bit of the nanosilver gel on her finger and rubbed it across the child's closed eyelid. The next day she was fine. **Obviously, as always, no claims are made by Harry that the nanosilver was the cause of her getting better. Precious Waters™ Nanosilver is FDA approved only as an immune system support.**

There is another instance of a 4-year-old boy badly burning his hand on and between the first finger and thumb when he put his hand on a hot outdoor camping grill and kept it there while he froze in fear. His grandmother poured the nanosilver on it while he was screaming in intense pain, and in 20 minutes he was just whimpering. The wound was left to the open air, and she poured more on occasionally. By the morning he was much improved. By the 4th day, she said you could not tell he had been burned.

This same woman took several of her grandchildren on a camping tour in a big recreational vehicle, and they all came down with what was probably a virus of some sort. They were all vomiting and had diarrhea. Now usually adults catch such a virus too, as any parent of school-age children will attest. In this case, though, she and her son-in-law, both of whom take the nanosilver regularly as a preventive, did not get sick. She attributes that to the nanosilver, which is only her opinion. Harry of course makes no claims.

## Vietnam Vets Should Know This

A 70-year-old Vietnam vet exposed to Agent Orange had severe actinic keratosis on his arms. His skin was scaly, rough and fire-engine red according to his wife. He had bleeding blisters. This is the most common form of pre-cancer. She did not want him to use the fluorouracil cream, the most common treatment, because it also destroys healthy cells, she said, when I spoke with her today.

Three weeks ago she started spraying his arms twice a day with the spray gel, which is specially formulated to penetrate the skin. At the start, being a skeptical RN, she didn't really think it would help all that much. To her surprise, the affected area quickly showed no more raised areas that are symptoms of actinic keratosis, and after using three bottles of the spray gel over three weeks, she says his right arm looked almost normal. His left arm was worse because it got more sun exposure from driving, but it too is improving dramatically.

As an aside, his younger brother, also exposed to Agent Orange in Vietnam, had the same condition, but not as severe. Still, the skin was itchy and inflamed, and the skin was rough. He applied the gel spray one evening, and the next day he claimed his skin was as smooth as a baby's. He said he couldn't believe it. While it's doubtful it was that smooth, he immediately bought three more bottles! Harry is happy about that, but makes no claims that the gel spray helped either brother.

## Fever Blisters & Rashes Disappear While Using Nanosilver

Fever blisters, also known as cold sores and oral herpes, are caused by the herpes simplex virus. They are very contagious and can commonly be transmitted from one person to another simply by kissing, so it is very common. A California man in his 60s had been bothered by them for some time. They were not only physically painful but also socially embarrassing. Literature says the sores usually heal in two or three weeks, but the virus remains, so they can recur regularly.

This man started taking nanosilver almost two months ago, and they disappeared almost immediately. He has had no problems since then. **Just as significant, he had been bothered for a long time by skin rashes on his arms, head and face, (some related to previous skin cancers) and these also either diminished dramatically or disappeared.** As a preventive, both he and his wife take a teaspoon of nanosilver once a day, though he isn't sure they need to. **As always, no claims are made.**

**Precious Waters™ Nanosilver is FDA approved only as an immune system support.**

# Chapter 14: Stories From Harry's Family

As you'd expect, Harry's family members are big fans of Precious Waters™ nanosilver. Here are just a few stories recounting times they used it themselves or provided it to someone they knew.

### 3rd Degree Burns – No Pain

Harry Watson's daughter-in-law Mary is a Registered Nurse and has seen a lot of medical situations over the years, including burns and rashes. Recently Dave, a fellow in his 30s who works with her son Cody, forgot that he was working with heated metal and reached down to pick it up, severely burning three of his fingertips.

Naturally he went to the Emergency Room in the nearest hospital as soon as possible, where they told him these were 3rd degree burns and gave him pain medications. He went home and to deal with the extreme pain he tried putting his fingertips on things like frozen vegetables, but he had to remove them often. He was in so much pain when he removed them that he was in tears, and asked Cody if he could think of anything that might help him. He was desperate.

Cody at that moment thought about Precious Waters™ gel spray. He called Mary, and she immediately sprayed enough gel into a sandwich-size plastic bag to allow the fingertips to be soaked in it. Cody picked up the bag and brought it to Dave, who stuck his fingertips into the gel for 7 minutes.

"What's in that stuff?" was Dave's reaction when he removed his fingertips and felt absolutely no pain. The next morning he was shocked to see how much better his fingertips looked. He continued to soak them occasionally over the next couple of days and at no time did he feel any further pain.

The doctors at the ER had told him it might take a long time to heal, which is why it is so remarkable that, after just 4 days, he already had light pink new skin covering the fingertips, never experienced any more pain, and totally healed in a short time. Nice coincidence, but no claims.

**Severe Diaper Rash**

In another recent situation Mary's 7-month-old great-granddaughter was teething and also developed a fiery red diaper rash. The mother's pediatrician suggested that perhaps Monistat, used by adult women for yeast infections, might help because such rashes are often caused by yeast.

Mary decided that first they might try spraying the Precious Waters™ nanosilver gel over the baby's vaginal area to see if it would help. They did so, then put the baby to bed. She slept seven hours, and when she awoke, the fiery redness was totally gone. By the next day, it was virtually totally healed.

Mary looked up some medical information online and found that since such rashes are often caused by yeast, a fungus, and various forms of silver can apparently kill fungus, she concluded this is probably why the healing occurred so quickly. That's only her conclusion though, and as always, no claims are made that the gel spray heals anything.

## Harry's Daughter Recovers from Dangerous Shingles on Her Scalp

Harry's daughter Theresa who lives in California recently developed a severe, painful case of Shingles on her scalp and forehead, dangerously close to her right eye. The doctor was concerned that she might lose sight in her right eye.

She started taking "strong" doses of the Precious Waters™ nanosilver water and also used the gel spray, both 3 to 4 times a day. She started feeling better right away, and after 3 days she no longer felt sick. After two weeks all symptoms were almost gone entirely and she had no pain.

Another happy coincidence! No cause and effect implied.

# Chapter 15: Some Serious Science for Silver... & If You're Hesitant...

Most chapters in this book are anecdotes about the happy coincidences of people who take Precious Waters™ and/or use the spray gel, and seem to get better. This chapter, however, is about some serious science supporting the notion that silver has infection-fighting properties unique among metals. If a medical doctor has told you not to try nanosilver as you are undergoing treatment for cancer, it is important for you to be aware of the following information.

Dr. Robert O. Becker was a respected orthopedic surgeon and prolific researcher who pioneered breakthroughs in applying electricity and electromagnetic treatments for tissue regeneration, and was twice nominated for the Nobel Prize. His first book, *The Body Electric,* published in 1985, is a classic in the field, and his second book, *Cross Currents,* published in 1990, details the promise of electromedicine and the perils of electropollution.

On pages 163-166 of *Cross Currents,* he summarizes a study of the biological effects of different kinds of metallic electrodes. He knew that the ions of metals are positive, so that positive voltage on the electrode repels them, and they are then pushed, or driven, into the tissues. This results in a voltage field containing large numbers of positive metal ions that can chemically react with membranes of living cells.

He suspected that this combination of an electric-voltage field and reactive metal ions might have unique effects on cells, so he and his team tested the effects of a variety of metallic electrodes on several different bacteria in culture, at voltage levels from very small to just above electrolysis level. Above the electrolysis level, the positive metal electrodes killed all bacteria, *but they would also have killed any human cells.* **Only the silver anode killed all bacteria at voltages that would be harmless to humans.**

He pointed out they had simply rediscovered what was known for centuries, that silver killed bacteria. But previous clinical applications used either silver foil or compounds, which didn't penetrate the tissues, and when antibiotics were discovered, clinical uses for silver as an antibiotic were discarded.

At the time of Dr. Becker's experiments nanosilver, engineered silver consistently producing nano-scale silver, whose particles are small enough to enter cell membranes, did not yet exist. And Precious Waters™ is *positively electrically charged.* So it can do what was impossible for silver foil or compounds to accomplish.

When Dr. Becker then conducted tests on patients, he learned that the electrically generated silver ion (equivalent to today's electrically charged nano-scale particles in Precious Waters™) was doing more than killing bacteria; it was also causing major growth stimulation of tissues in the wound.

Amazingly, he and his team found that the human fibroblast cells in the area *dedifferentiated, so they were able to multiply at a great rate and produce large numbers of primitive, embryonic cells in the wound. These in turn were able to differentiate into whatever types of cells were needed to heal the wound.* **They were turning on regeneration in human tissues**... something previously thought impossible.

This led to the question, would the silver ions dedifferentiate human cancer cells? A lack of funds prevented further exploration; however, they did find that some human cancer cells in culture appeared to dedifferentiate when exposed to the silver ions.

One of Dr. Becker's patients with severe chronic bone infection and an associated cancer in the wound, refused amputation and insisted on being treated with the silver technique. After 3 months the infection was under control **and the cancer cells in the wound appeared to have changed back to normal.** After eight years, when Dr. Becker last heard from him, he was still cancer-free.

Dr. Becker pointed out that this patient's treatment was an **electrochemical** treatment, not simply electrical. He surmised that the silver ion was shaped so as to connect to a receptor group on the surface of the cancer cell membrane, and that once that connection was made, an electrical-charge transfer sends a signal to the nucleus of the cancer cell that activates the primitive-type genes, **and the cell dedifferentiates.**

A highly respected oncologist at a major cancer center told me, in answer to my question, that cancer cells can never become normal cells. That is probably what 100% of oncologists would say, but it's also likely they are not aware of Dr. Becker, his books, or his research because oncology has traditionally focused on chemo, radiation and surgery. Electromagnetic or electrochemical modalities are not something practitioners are generally aware of. At the very least, as some of the anecdotes in this book show, taking Precious Waters™ while taking chemotherapy seems to do no harm.

### Silver & Antibiotics—1000x more power?

A 6/21/13 *Los Angeles Times* article makes the point that small amounts of silver added to antibiotics can make the antibiotics up to 1000x more powerful in mice. Beyond showing the potential impact of silver, it raises the question: when doctors administering chemotherapy tell a person not to take nanosilver, are they giving the best advice? The article reported on a study published in the respected publication *Science Translational Medicine.* News of it was picked up in several national media.

### What's So Special About Precious Waters™ Nanosilver?

Some people, when they hear about Precious Waters™, note that nanosilver is nothing new and that it has been around for years, widely used in the U.S. and Asia. They assume there are no significant differences between Precious Waters™ and other types of nanosilver. Harry

Watson cannot speak for other types of nanosilver, but if you are thinking of taking or recommending Precious Waters™, it is important for you to understand its properties and how it is manufactured. The processes to make it are proprietary, and result in some extraordinary properties.

## Large Surface Area in Proportion to Mass

When the nanoparticles are formed, they have a large surface area in proportion to the mass of the entire particle. When this happens, its ability to kill pathogens becomes extremely powerful in relation to its size. In Precious Waters™, all the particles also fall within a very narrow size range, resulting in consistency. The manufacturing process is one of the first to consistently produce a solution with a majority of silver particle size distribution in the sub 10 nanometer range. This is considered the "sweet spot" for the ability to neutralize harmful pathogens.

## Special Type of Electrical Charge Attracts Pathogens

The Precious Waters™ manufacturing process is unique. Silver in its native ionic state has a +2 valence; in other words it is positively charged and more so than most metals. The manufacturing process that creates the Precious Waters™ solution optimizes the particle size, its bio-availability and its bio-activity, resulting in a pure solution of just water and silver particles at 10ppm concentration. It accomplishes this under a process that uses proprietary electro-chemical techniques.

By creating a supplement in which the highly positively charged silver particles easily disassociate from the water and can travel throughout the body's system at the cellular level, you have a mechanism that is acting on the same level as the pathogens. There are several theories on how the positively charged silver particles actually disrupt or destroy the pathogens and stimulate some of the body's repair functions, but from a layman's standpoint the normally negatively charged pathogens are drawn to the positively charged silver particles, which are able to neutralize or modify the pathogens' behavior.

With this knowledge in hand, it becomes easier to understand why there are so many anecdotes about people taking Precious Waters™ who improve dramatically, sometimes from what would otherwise be fatal diseases. It also becomes easier to understand, for example, why the clinical trials in Kenya showed such remarkable results for HIV patients when Precious Waters™ was taken along with drugs.

**What's New & Not New**

If someone tells you that they already use nanosilver, or that it is nothing new, they are right that the category itself is not new. But the use of Precious Waters™ has not been widespread to this point, and the clinical trial results in Kenya are new as of the last few years. This means, whatever people have in mind when they speak of "knowing all about nanosilver," it is very likely they do not know about the properties of Precious Waters™.

**If You're Hesitant About Taking Precious Waters™**

Many people are hesitant to try silver supplements and that is understandable given that an internet search can reveal some seemingly shady operations. As with any product, some suppliers are only interested in a "quick buck," while others might be well intentioned, but offer products that are not safe if misused.

Doctors too will often discourage people from taking any supplements, including minerals like silver. Often this is because they haven't heard of it before, don't know anything about it, and might therefore be concerned about liability. Oncologists will often discourage people with cancer from taking it because they don't want it to interfere with the chemo or other prescribed treatment regimen they are administering.

By sharing the anecdotes and other information in this book, my aim is to make readers aware of a supplement that has a long history of success in supporting people's natural immune system. Each person can then take charge of their own health, make choices accordingly, and where they consider it prudent, supplement whatever regimen they are undergoing.

As noted, Precious Waters™ is allowed for sale only as a dietary supplement, so claims cannot be made that it is effective against disease. On the other hand, as noted earlier, studies conducted in 2006 by scientists at Pennsylvania State University and Arizona State University documented the fact that Precious Waters™ nanosilver poses no harm when consumed.

Separate lab tests in 2007 conducted by others

showed its effectiveness against HIV and Avian Influenza, and the fact that when it was combined with 19 different antibiotics, it improved their effectiveness. They also noted the safe use of silver as an orally consumed preventive agent, demonstrated and supported by reports from the EPA and the US Department of Health and Human Services, where in a 76-week long study, dogs that inhaled silver showed activity in the lung in one hour, with 90% of the silver carried to the liver by the blood within six hours.

In other words, **it was proven to be non-toxic to animals even in quantities that would be far greater than a human would ever ingest.**

In addition to this scientific input, you can take into consideration the stories in this book about people who have taken Precious Waters™ and at the same time coincidentally recovered from diseases and illnesses ranging from cancer and malaria to endometriosis, HIV, TB and several other diseases caused by a virus, bacteria or fungus.

The journal *Molecules* published an article in 2011 that summarized the effectiveness of nanosilver against many viruses and bacteria. The article contains glowing comments about the effectiveness of nanosilver in killing viruses and bacteria.

You can also take into consideration the fact that Precious Waters™ is nonionic and not colloidal. It is converted by the body into ionic form only after ingestion, and therefore does not result in silver chloride or other unwanted salts precipitating out.

Currently, **over half a dozen doctors around the country order Precious Waters™ from Harry,** and one of them wants to order in quantities large enough so that he can private-label it for his patients. And let's not forget the results of carefully monitored and certified **clinical trials conducted in Kenya** noted earlier.

Each person will make up their own mind as to whether they want to try Precious Waters™. That is as it should be. The main challenge Harry has encountered over the years is that some people find negative information on the internet about possible toxicity of silver. That information is *totally irrelevant to Precious Waters™.*

As they should, many people go to their doctors for an opinion. The problem is, most of the doctors are not aware of even the general category of nanosilver and will reject it out of hand, knowing nothing about it. This is not a problem when people recover from their illness anyway, but it is heartbreaking to learn of people who died after conventional treatment, or who suffered from roughly the same condition that others recovered from after taking Precious Waters™. As noted, no cause and effect relationship is claimed, but it is sad to hear of these cases.

It is vital to take into account all input from medical professionals you trust, but it is also important to determine how much they know about silver in general, about Precious Waters™ in particular, and to consider all the input mentioned here.

# Chapter 16: Precious Waters™ Label and Cost Comparison

Here is the copy of the Precious Waters™ label. As noted previously, **no claims are made that it directly affects any diseases whatsoever.**

### PRECIOUS WATERS™
Advanced Nano-Silver Dietary Supplement

- Immune System Support
- Patented Process
- Scientifically Tested
- 10 ppm Silver Solution

   8 fl. oz. (236 ml)

Suggested use:

Adults: 1 teaspoon once or twice daily
Children: ¼ to ½ teaspoon once daily

WARNING: If you are pregnant, nursing, have any reaction to trace minerals or if you have any chronic or recurring symptoms or illness, please consult a health care professional before using this product.

KEEP OUT OF REACH OF CHILDREN

Store at room temperature.
Keep out of direct sunlight.
Do not use if seal is broken.

This product is a dietary supplement. It is not
intended to diagnose, treat, cure, or prevent any
disease. The FDA has not evaluated these statements.

**Supplement Facts**
Serving Size: 1 tsp. (5ml)
Servings per container: 48
Amount Per Serving
Purified Silver 50 mcg(*)
*Daily Value not established.
10 ppm Silver Solution

Other ingredients: Deionized Water
Contains no artificial ingredients, preservatives or
additives.

Manufactured for and Distributed by:
Trinity Silver Solutions, LLC
PO Box 406
Weaverville CA 96093
Tel. 530-739-8600

(end of label copy)

## Cost of Drugs vs Cost of Precious Waters™
One of the positive things about Precious Waters™ is that
most people in the United States can easily afford it. It

might or might not help them, and Harry Watson never makes any claims, but many people have had strong recoveries from serious diseases at the same time they happened to be taking it, and a person risks very little financially for trying it.

Its low cost is in sharp contrast to a 2014 Bloomberg News article which points out that, for a variety of reasons, the price of 73 drug brands increased 75% from 2007 to 2014. It recounts several instances where new drugs can cost in the hundreds of thousands of dollars for total treatment, and mentions one specific instance where an older drug for multiple sclerosis that cost about $550 per injection in 2007, costs almost $1200 seven years later. Apparently, a drug loses revenues when competitors enter the market, so drug manufacturers will sometimes raise prices to make up for the lost revenues.

Without passing judgment on the justification for these price increases, the fact remains we are all stuck with higher prices for many drugs, especially those that treat serious diseases such as cancer, leukemia and diabetes. We are also faced with much greater uncertainty about whether those of us who need these drugs will be able to afford them or to get access to them under Medicare and Affordable Care Act restrictions and limitations. It is not a comforting thought.

Precious Waters™ is not a drug, and no claims are made that it can have any effect on any disease, despite the many interesting anecdotes in this book. Neither does it require the huge costs of research, development and clinical trials that drugs must go through, with only a fraction of them proving to be winners. As noted, it is simply nano-sized highly engineered particles of silver in purified water, electrically charged in proprietary processes involving specific formulas for pressure, temperature, electrical charge and duration, so it is indeed complex. Still, it can be manufactured relatively inexpensively compared to drugs.

For the person who cannot get access to the expensive drugs required to treat his or her serious disease, and for those who have been told by medical doctors there is no more that can be done for them, it doesn't cost much to give Precious Waters™ a try, to see if perhaps the same happy coincidences that have occurred for others might also occur for them.

The same holds true even if the condition is not a serious one, as many anecdotes in this book indicate. Anything from a toothache to fever blisters might coincidentally disappear at the same time you happen to be taking Precious Waters™, and it doesn't cost much to find out.

# Chapter 17: So What Are We to Make of it All?

So there you have it. A number of anecdotes from the past year, testimonials from other years, the results of clinical trials in Kenya, and some scientific input. As stated *ad nauseum* in this book, the anecdotes are just that, nothing more, and no claims can be made about them. They are presented as interesting coincidences, nothing more.

Still, people can act on coincidences if they wish to. It has been frustrating for Harry Watson to learn of people who refuse to try Precious Waters™ and ultimately die, but each person makes his or her own decision about whether they want to try something that is allowed by the FDA to be sold only as a dietary supplement.

So why bother to write this book? Because if it's really this simple for a lot of people to experience dramatic improvements from infections and diseases, but they don't even try, it feels like a tragedy. Even if people use Precious Waters™ only as a supplement to conventional treatment, think of the tens of thousands of people it might help, not just in the U.S., but globally. What a shame it would be if the simple addition of this unique form of nanosilver to a treatment regimen could have helped. The hope is that someday, some of this information will filter through to people who can make a difference, and that some company or organization will begin to conduct trials in the U.S. that enable medical claims to be made for this wonderful product.

On the other hand, maybe it wouldn't prove out, but with all the anecdotal evidence piling up, and the results of the Kenyan clinical trials, I hope that at least one prominent cancer researcher in the U.S. will notice and be curious enough to conduct some experiments.

Perhaps most researchers mistakenly assume that today's oligodynamic, highly engineered, positively electrochemically charged Precious Waters™ nano-scale silver is no different from the colloidal silver of a decade ago. I hope this book makes them aware of the advances that have been made.

This book was also written to make people aware of all these coincidences, in the hope that they will consider these stories when deciding whether they want to try Precious Waters™. As noted, some people use only the nanosilver; many use it with baking soda to make their system more alkaline; and some take it while receiving chemotherapy, either letting their doctors know or not.

If you suffer from a condition that conventional treatment doesn't seem to help, please know you have my best wishes for a speedy recovery no matter what you decide! Thanks for considering this input. If you want to contact Susan or Mark, please visit the website at www.preciouswatersinc.com or call them on 530-739-8600.

# About the Author

Dan McAneny is a 5x cancer survivor. At the end of 2006 he learned he had two serious cancers. One of them, non-Hodgkin's B-cell lymphoma, kept coming back in different places, first surrounding a kidney and then in his stomach and groin. He was fine after two years of chemo and radiation at Duke University Medical Center in 2007-08, ending in November 2008.

He stayed healthy until the fall of 2011, when the lymphoma returned with a vengeance in his stomach. Once again, the chemo did its job and he was better by the end of the year. Other than a failed bone marrow transplant procedure two months later, that was the last treatment Dan had, and he is today quite healthy.

None of Dan's treatments involved nanosilver, but the cocktails the doctors used at Duke and Moffitt Cancer Center in Tampa often included metals, including platinum. That's why Dan was predisposed to accept Harry Watson's experience with silver just as Harry described it. His motivation was to assist in Harry's quest to build awareness of Precious Waters™ among people with cancer, HIV, TB or any other disease caused by a virus, bacteria or fungus.

Dan recently retired as a disability consultant. In that capacity, he was compensated by insurance companies to help people on long-term disability start or buy businesses. He directed interested clients in the required research and then created business plans for those whose businesses seemed viable, or if not, advised them to explore other options. He and his wife Pat now live in Sarasota, Florida. They have five children and eleven grandchildren. Dan has written several other books: two for people on disability who want to get back into action, and eight on his 50-year-long study of the afterlife and its positive implications for happier daily living.

Made in the USA
San Bernardino, CA
04 August 2020

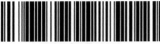